You Can Fight Cancer

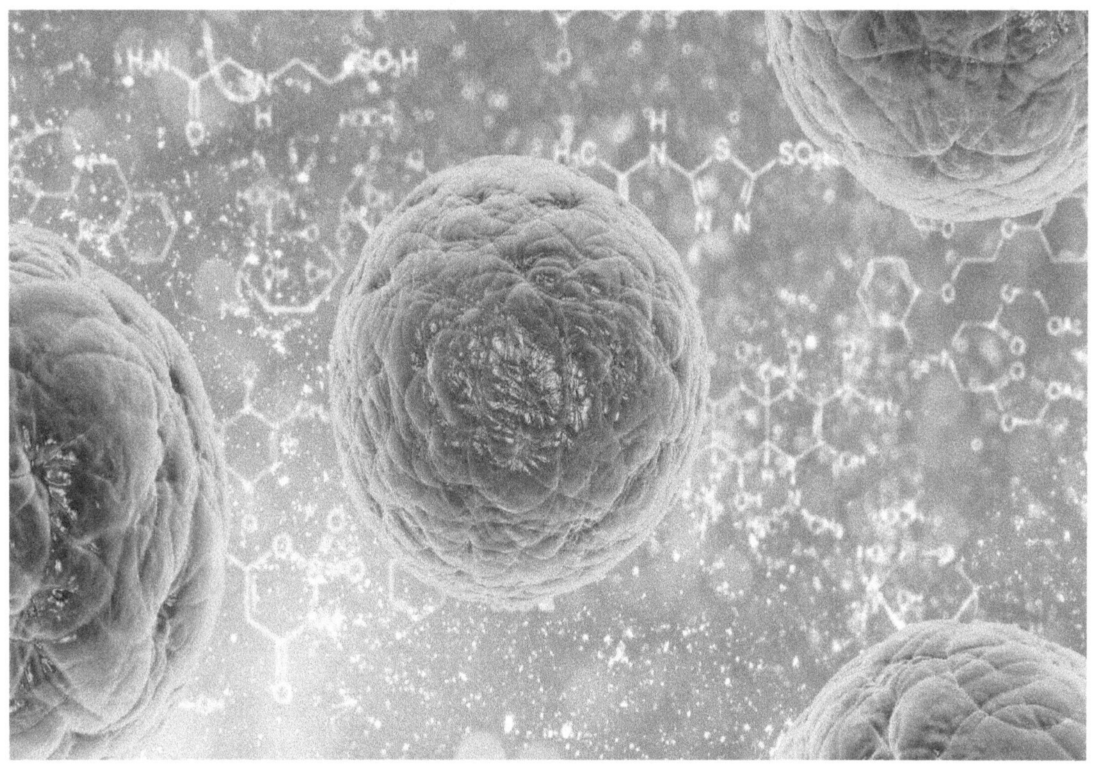

An Inspiration to Natural Healing For Cancer Survivors (With Oncologist Approved Metabolic And Nutritional Approach)

Caroline Johnson

TABLE OF CONTENTS

Introduction

It all started with a routine check-up, where Ellie was diagnosed with cancer. She was devastated and felt like her whole world had come crashing down. The thought of undergoing chemotherapy and losing her hair was terrifying to her. She felt angry, scared, and alone.

Her doctor reassured her that the cancer was in its early stages and with proper treatment, she had a good chance of recovery. But Ellie couldn't shake off the feeling of fear and hopelessness. She couldn't imagine living with cancer for the rest of her life.

After feeling sad and accepting to face reality, Ellie decided to sit up and take the necessary actions concerning her situation. She began to carry out research concerning cancer and also hear from other people who has been through her current stage of life. She began to read and follow guidelines and treatment advice from experts in the health field and also read about cancer survivors who has battled with cancer and won.

The book also provided information about different treatment options and how one's mindset plays a crucial role in the healing process. Ellie was determined to apply the lessons she learned from the book to her own journey.

She started taking better care of her physical and mental health. She went for walks in the park, practiced meditation, and started eating a well-balanced diet. She also connected with support groups and joined an online community for cancer patients.

Slowly but surely, Ellie's perspective towards her illness started to shift. Instead of feeling defeated, she felt a sense of empowerment. She realized that she had the power to fight and overcome cancer. The book had given her a glimmer of hope that she thought was lost.

As she went for her chemotherapy sessions, Ellie would take the book with her and read a few pages before each session. It gave her the strength and courage she needed to keep going.

After months of treatment and a lot of ups and downs, Ellie received the news she had been waiting for – she was cancer-free. Her recovery was not just a physical one; it was a transformation of her mind and soul.

Ellie went on to share her story with others and even started a support group…

Dealing with cancer can be challenging. We understand the journey through this battle and have had patients fight and recover from this battle. It's important you know that "You are not the first to have this problem" others have experienced this and conquered. We are here with you in this journey through cancer, and we look forward to having you as one of our numerous cancer survivors who has fought and conquered.

This book contains all you need to stay strong and ready for the journey ahead of you, the emotional, psychological and physical well-being you need for this journey and also nutritional approach of fighting this enemy.

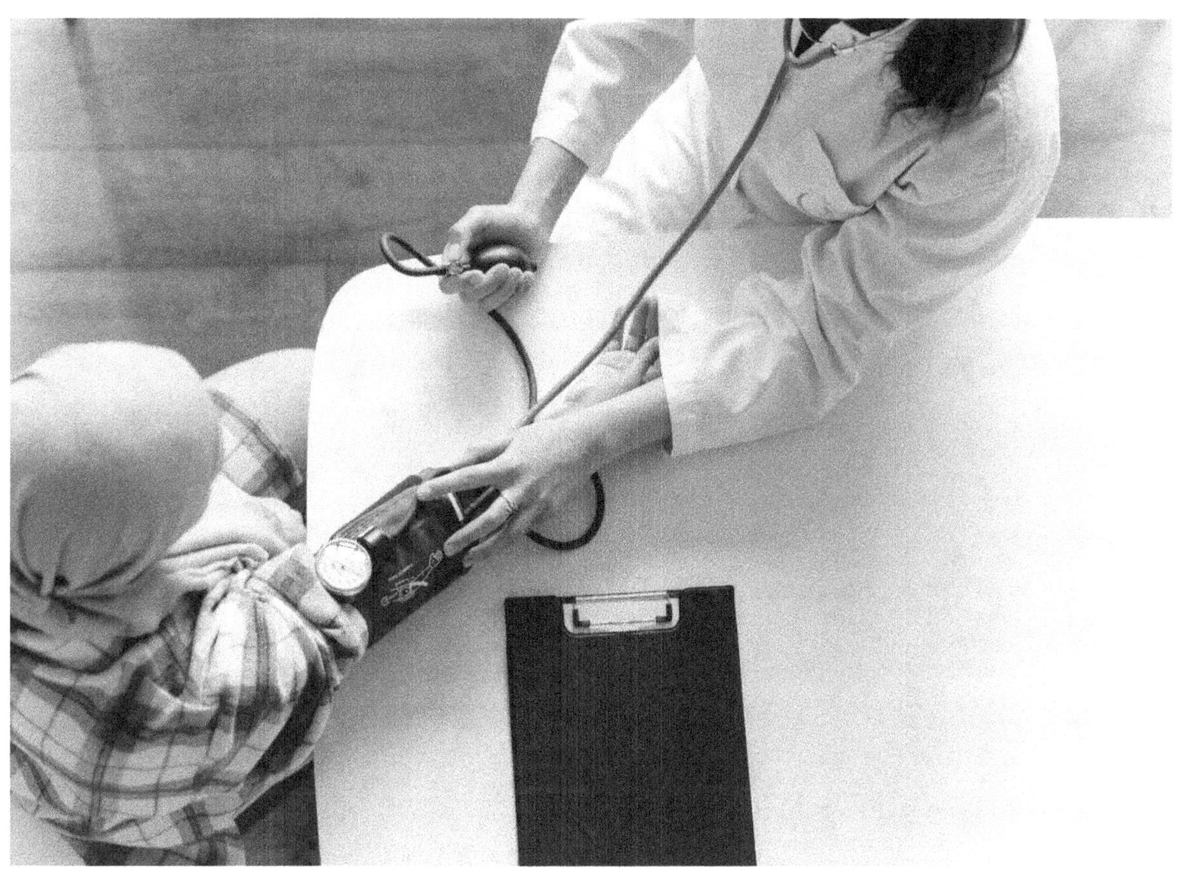

Chapter 1: The Breaking News: Just Realizing you have cancer

The world stops spinning when the words "you have cancer" echo in your ears. Everything else becomes a blur as your mind struggles to comprehend the magnitude of this news. It's a surreal moment when the doctor delivers the diagnosis, and you feel like you're watching someone else's life play out before your eyes. But then it hits you, this is your reality now. The shock slowly gives way to a flood of emotions. Fear, sadness, anger, confusion - they all swirl around inside you, threatening to consume you.

You try to hold back tears, not wanting to break down in front of the doctor, but it's no use. The tears fall freely as the weight of the news bears down on you. Questions start flooding your mind. How did this happen? How long have I had it? Will I survive? What about my family? It's overwhelming, and there are no easy answers. You try to focus on the doctor's voice, to understand the treatment options, but it feels like you're underwater. The words are muffled, and you struggle to make sense of it all.

As you leave the doctor's office, the flood of emotions continues. You feel the weight of the news like a heavy burden on your shoulders. The world around you suddenly seems darker and more uncertain. The things that once seemed important now pale in comparison to the battle you're about to face. As you call your loved ones to tell them the news, your heart breaks at the thought of their reactions.

How do you tell your spouse, your parents, your children that you have cancer? How will they handle it? And then the thoughts turn inward. Guilt for not taking better care of yourself and catching it sooner. Frustration for the unknowns and the long road ahead. Regret for all the things you wish you had done differently. But amidst all the turmoil, there is also a glimmer of hope. The doctor said there are treatment options, and there is a chance for survival. You cling to this hope like a lifeline, knowing that it's all you have. In the days and weeks that follow, you begin to adjust to this new reality.

It's not easy, and there are moments of despair and fear, but you find strength in the support of your loved ones. You also learn to lean on the incredible community of cancer survivors who have walked this path before you. You realize that this journey will be one of the greatest challenges you will ever face, but you are determined to strive and not just give up so soon. The news may have shattered your world, but it has also made you appreciate the fragility of life and to embrace every moment with the ones you love. You also understand that cancer does not define you. You are still the same person you were before the diagnosis, with hopes and dreams and the will to fight.

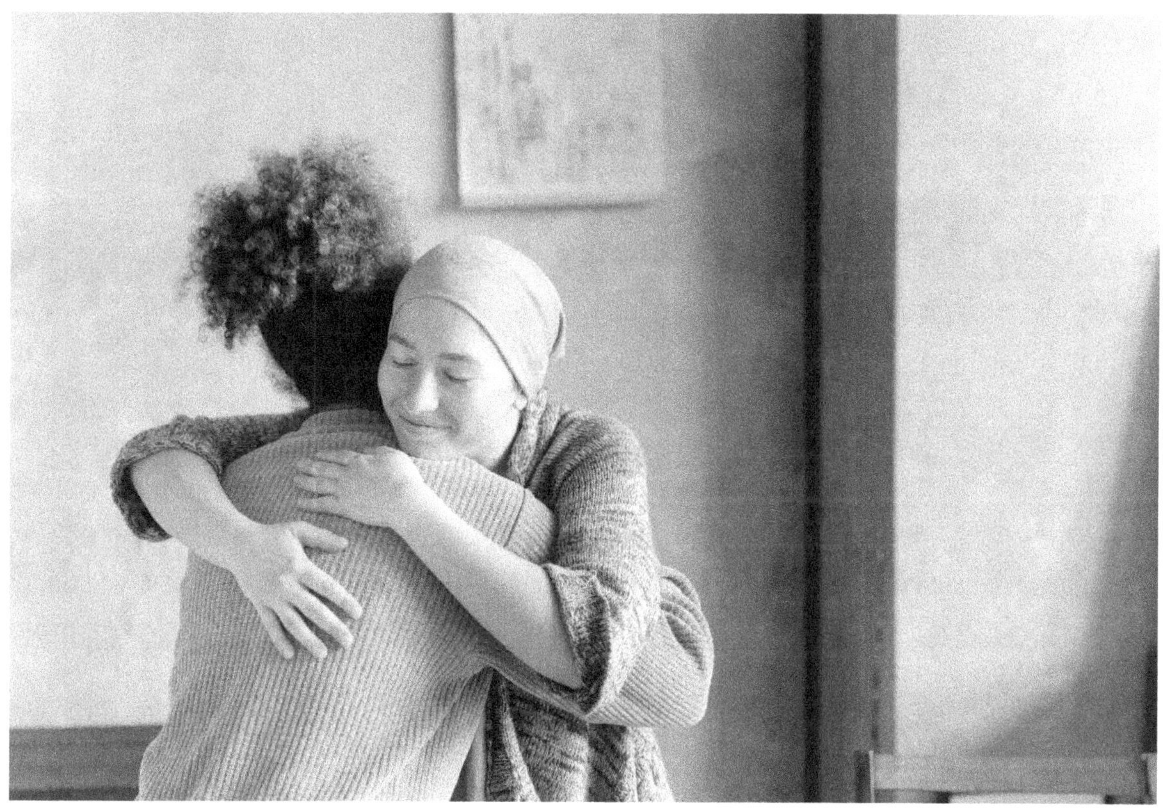

Chapter 2: Being patient in the waiting room: Coping with Cancer

After finding out you have cancer then what next? It important you know that you need not to panic. It is of no doubt that you will have to adjust to somethings in other to be fit to beat this disease called cancer. Not only does cancer take a physical toll on the body, but it also has a profound impact on one's emotional and mental well-being. Coping with cancer can be a difficult and challenging journey, but with the right strategies and support, it is possible to live a fulfilling life despite the disease. In this chapter, we will discuss some techniques and tips on how to cope with cancer and live a better quality of life.

1. Educate Yourself: The first step in coping with cancer is to educate yourself about the disease. It's essential to understand your diagnosis and treatment options, including the potential side effects. This will help you make informed decisions and be prepared for what lies ahead. Additionally, do your research and learn about support groups and resources available in your community. Having knowledge about your condition will empower you and give you a sense of control over your situation.

2. Build a Strong Support System: It's crucial to have a strong support network while dealing with cancer be with people who love and care for you. Lean on your family, friends, and loved ones for emotional and practical support. They can be a source of comfort, and their presence can lift your spirits on the tough days

3. Take Good Care of Yourself: While treating cancer, it's important to maintain a healthy diet and lifestyle. Eating well can help you feel stronger and cope with the side effects of treatment. Incorporate plenty of fruits and vegetables, whole grains, and lean proteins into your diet. Avoid processed and sugary foods, which can contribute to fatigue and other symptoms. Also, try to get enough rest and exercise regularly, as it can help boost your energy levels and improve your overall well-being. Do well to see your doctor before starting any exercise routine.

4. Practice Mindfulness and Relaxation Techniques: Dealing with cancer can be emotionally draining, and it's essential to take care of your mental health as well. Practicing mindfulness and relaxation techniques such as meditation, yoga, or deep breathing can help reduce stress, anxiety, and improve your overall outlook. You can also try activities that you enjoy, such as listening to music, reading, or painting. These activities can help you relax and provide a much-needed distraction from thinking and stressing too much.

As a cancer patient, you need to also know that you are not alone in the cancer fight. You are loved and they is a whole community out there waiting to see you get through this terribly tough time.

5. Seek Professional Support: As a cancer patient, you need to also know that you are not alone in the cancer fight. You are loved and they is a whole community out there waiting to see you get through this terribly tough time. It's completely normal to feel overwhelmed, anxious, and depressed while dealing with cancer. If your emotions are becoming too difficult to manage, don't hesitate to seek professional support. Professional counselors and therapists can provide you with specialized techniques and tools to help you cope with your emotional distress.

6. Find a Sense of Purpose: Cancer can often make you feel like your life has been put on hold, and it's easy to lose your sense of purpose. However, finding a sense of purpose, whether it's a new hobby or volunteering, can give you a sense of fulfillment and a reason to keep going. It can also provide you with a positive outlook and a sense of hope for the future.

7. Stay Positive: Maintaining a positive attitude can be challenging, but it's essential for coping with cancer. Try to focus on the present and make the most of each day. Keep yourself motivated by setting small goals and celebrating your achievements, however small they may seem. Surround yourself with positivity and try to avoid negative thoughts and people who bring you down.

Join a Support Group: Connecting with other cancer patients who are going through similar experiences can provide you with a sense of belonging and comfort. Joining a support group can also help you learn from others and share your own experiences. These groups can also provide practical tips and resources for coping with cancer.

9. Be Kind to Yourself: Living with cancer can be physically, emotionally, and mentally challenging. It's essential to be kind to yourself and practice self-care. Allow yourself to rest when you need it, and don't push yourself too hard.

10. Be Open and Honest: Many cancer patients tend to isolate themselves and push away their loved ones out of fear or shame. However, it's crucial to be open and honest about how you feel and what you need from your support system. Communicate your emotions and concerns to your loved ones and healthcare team.

11. Creative outlets: Engaging in creative activities such as painting, writing, or playing an instrument can serve as a distraction from cancer-related stressors, and also serve as an emotional outlet to express feelings that may be difficult to put into words.

Coping with cancer is a journey that requires strength, resilience, and support. It's normal to experience a range of emotions while dealing with cancer, but by following the tips mentioned above, you can learn to manage your emotions and live a fulfilling Life.

Chapter 3: Breaking The Stigma: Living with cancer and coping with fear

Cancer is a word that can strike fear into the hearts of anyone who hears it. It is a disease that has been plaguing humankind for centuries, and despite advancements in medical technology and treatments, it is still a source of anxiety, pain, and suffering for millions of people across the globe.

The stigma surrounding cancer is deeply ingrained in our culture and is fueled by misinformation, fear, and prejudice. Many people view cancer as a death sentence and those who have it as weak or deserving of their illness.

Many cancer patients feel pressure to keep their illness a secret or downplay its severity, for fear of being judged or treated differently. That feeling is understandable, but you do not have to feel sorry. You should not allow yourself be an object of pity or give chance for the outside world to shape who you are and how much value you hold. This can make it difficult for you to talk about your feelings and needs, making the already difficult journey of living with cancer even harder.

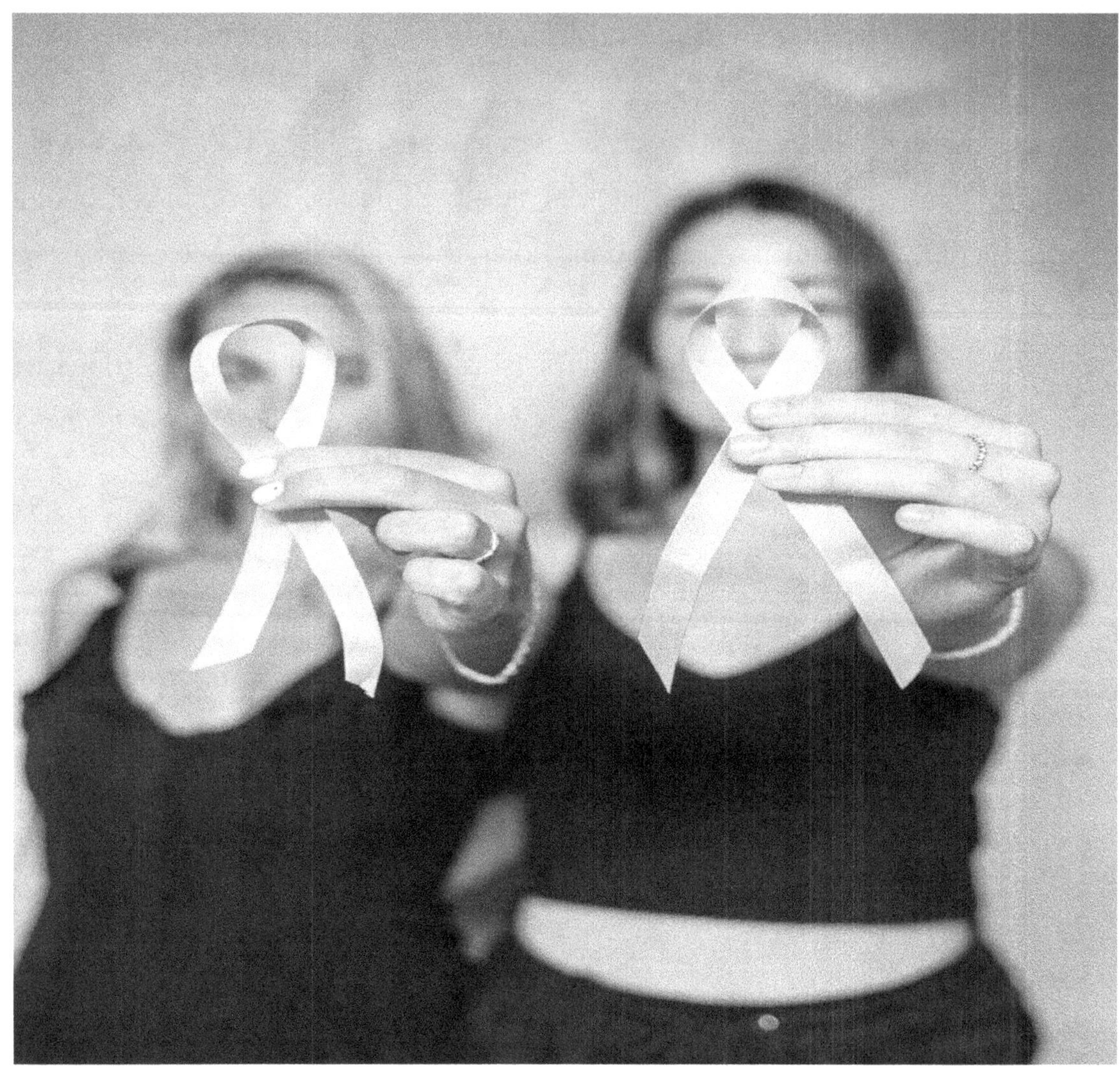

Breaking the stigma surrounding cancer is crucial for your well-being as a cancer patient. It is essential to recognize that cancer is not a punishment or a sign of weakness. It is a complex illness that can affect anyone, regardless of age, gender, or lifestyle. By breaking these mindset, you can create a more understanding and understanding relationships with love ones and family. You do not have to be afraid, you are not alone in the stigma fight against cancer.

There are awareness campaigns and organized Communities also taking action for stopping stigma against cancer patients. and creating awareness to ensure that the society supports and uplifts cancer patients rather than shaming and ostracizing them. These communities also increase awareness and education about cancer. By providing accurate and up-to-date information about the disease, we can dispel myths and misconceptions and replace them with facts and understanding. This can help reduce fear and create a more informed and supportive community for cancer patients.

In addition, supporting and uplifting cancer patients can also help break the stigma. Instead of pity or judgment, we should offer empathy, compassion, and practical support. Simple acts of kindness, such as offering a helping hand or listening ear, can make a significant difference in the lives of those living with cancer. By being there for them, we can show that cancer is not something to be ashamed of, but an illness that deserves empathy and support. It is also crucial to promote a positive and empowering narrative around cancer.

Rather than focusing solely on the negative aspects, we should highlight stories of resilience, strength, and hope. By showcasing the experiences of cancer survivors and the progress made in cancer research, we can transform the way society perceives and talks about cancer.

In conclusion, breaking the stigma surrounding cancer is crucial for the well-being of those living with the disease. By increasing awareness, promoting empathy and understanding, and uplifting cancer patients, we can create a more supportive and compassionate society. Cancer may be a challenging and scary journey, but with the right support and a stigma-free environment, those living with it can find the strength and courage to face their fears and live fulfilling lives.

Read Related books by Caroline Johnson

https://mybook.to/Starve_breast_cancer

https://mybook.to/Teenage_Sexuality

https://mybook.to/Christmas_Recipe

Chapter 4: Cancer Is Not The End

Dear friend, I heard you have been diagnosed with cancer. I know this news must have been devastating and overwhelming for you and your loved ones. I want you to know that you are not alone in this journey, and there is hope.

I am writing this to encourage and inspire you to stay strong, have faith, and never lose hope. First and foremost, I want you to know that cancer does not define you. It may be a part of your life, but it does not define who you are as a person. You are so much more than the disease you are battling. You are a fighter, a warrior, and a survivor. You have the strength and determination to overcome this obstacle and come out even stronger.

I understand that cancer can be daunting, both physically and emotionally. The treatments may be exhausting, and the side effects can be tough, but you have to believe that they are working towards your recovery. Remember, it is a temporary phase, and it will pass. You have to keep pushing through it, even on the days when you feel like giving up. Take one day at a time, and celebrate each small victory.

Set realistic goals for yourself, and do not be too hard on yourself on the difficult days Surround yourself with positive and supportive people. Your family, friends, and caregivers are your biggest cheerleaders. They will provide the love, care, and support that you need to get through this. Do not be afraid to ask for help when you need it. Let them be there for you, and let them show you how much they care. Join a support group or connect with other cancer patients – these individuals will understand your struggles and can offer valuable advice and support.

It is also essential to take care of your emotional well-being. Cancer can take a toll on your mental health, and you may experience a range of emotions, including fear, anger, and sadness. It is okay to feel these emotions, but do not let them consume you. Find healthy ways to cope with your feelings, such as journaling, meditation, or talking to a therapist. Remember to be kind to yourself and practice self-care. Engage in activities you enjoy, and make time for yourself. You are deserving of love and care, especially during this difficult time. I want to remind you that cancer is not a death sentence.

Many people have fought and won the battle against cancer. Each cancer journey is unique, and yours will have its own set of challenges, but never lose hope. Believe in the power of positive thinking. Self-belief is a powerful tool in the fight against cancer. Our thoughts have the power to shape our reality, so focus on the good in your life. Celebrate your strengths and achievements, no matter how small they may seem. Surround yourself with positivity, whether it is through inspiring quotes, affirmations, or music. You can get through what ever obstacle that comes your way, be it mentally, Physically or emotionally. Read more on how to get over mental defeat and be strong to face life challenges on Grow your mind by Caroline Johnson

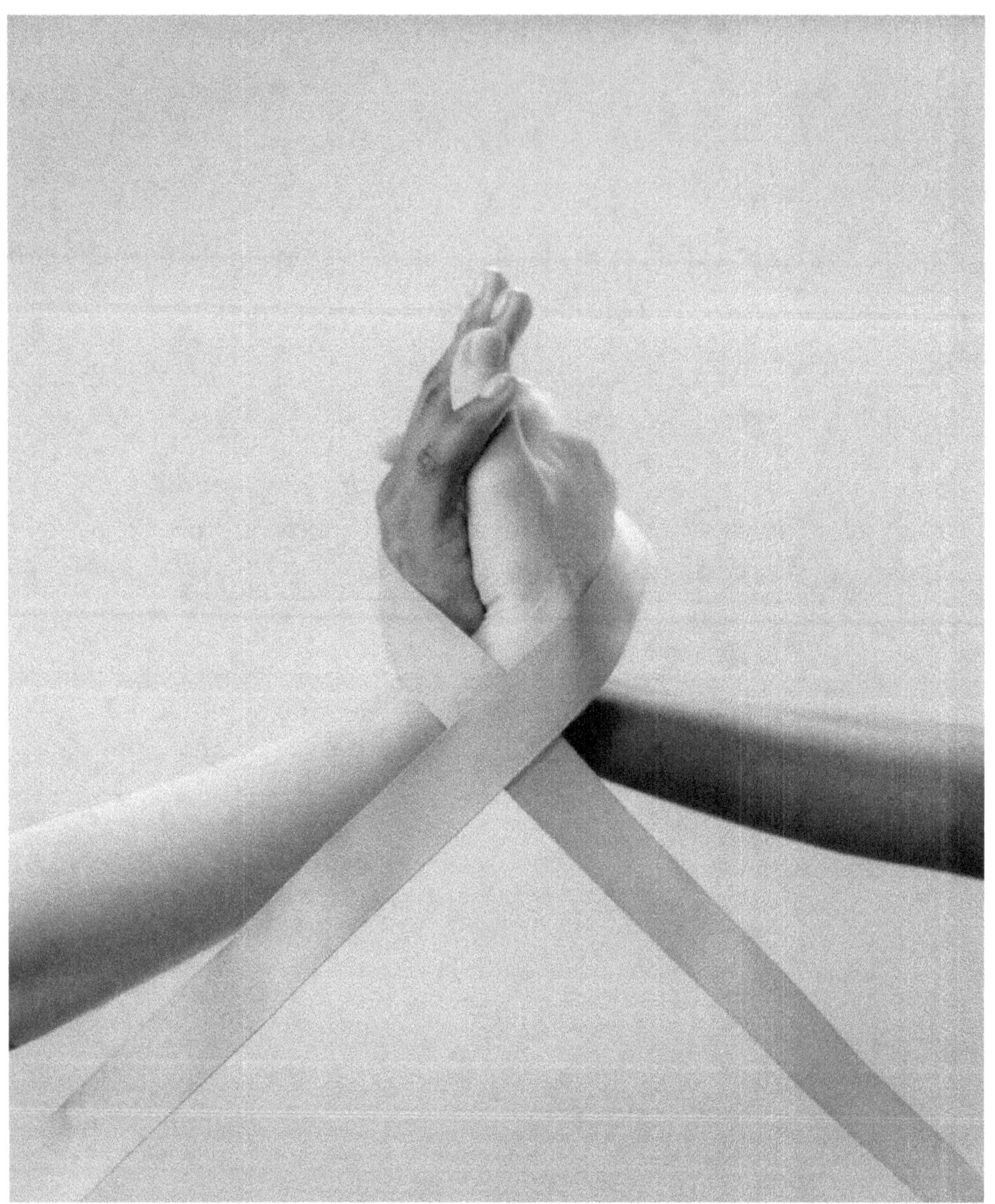

Remember to listen to your body and take care of it. Eat a healthy and balanced diet, as it will help to fuel your body and give you the energy you need to fight. Exercise regularly, even if it is just small movements in bed. Exercise has been proven to improve mood and reduce fatigue. Stay hydrated, and get enough rest to allow your body to heal. Finally, always hold on to hope. Believe in the strength of your body and the advancements in medical treatments.

Medical research and technology are constantly evolving, and new treatments and therapies are being discovered that are improving survival rates. Have faith that you will come out of this stronger and more resilient. In conclusion, dear friend, I want you to know that you are a fighter, and you can overcome this battle. Your journey may be tough, but you are tougher. Remember to stay positive, surround yourself with love and support, and take the cancer fight seriously.

Nutrition plays a crucial role in our overall health and well-being. This is especially true when it comes to preventing and fighting serious diseases like cancer. While there is no single food or nutrient that can completely prevent or cure cancer, following a healthy and balanced diet can help strengthen the body's immune system and reduce the risk of developing certain types of cancer.

Here are some of the various nutritional approaches that can help fight cancer:

1. Eat a plant-based diet: Eating a diet rich in fruits, vegetables, whole grains, and legumes is essential for overall health and can provide powerful protection against cancer. These foods are high in vitamins, minerals, antioxidants, and phytochemicals – all of which help boost the immune system and fight cancer-causing agents in the body. It is recommended to aim for at least 5 servings of fruits and vegetables per day.

2. Limit processed and red meats: Processed meats, such as bacon, hot dogs, and deli meats, have been linked to an increased risk of cancer. They contain nitrates and other preservatives that can damage cells and lead to cancer development. Red meats, such as beef, pork, and lamb, should also be consumed in moderation as they contain saturated fat, which has been linked to an increased risk of colon and other types of cancer. Instead of processed and red meats, opt for lean protein sources like fish, poultry, and plant-based proteins like beans and lentils.

3. Include anti-inflammatory foods: Inflammation is the body's natural response to injury and infection, but chronic inflammation has been linked to an increased risk of cancer. Including anti-inflammatory foods in your diet can help reduce this risk. These include fatty fish like salmon and tuna, leafy greens like spinach and kale, and colorful fruits like berries and cherries. These foods contain omega-3 fatty acids, antioxidants, and other nutrients that can help fight inflammation in the body.

4. Choose whole grains: Whole grains, such as brown rice, quinoa, and whole wheat, are excellent sources of fiber and other important nutrients. They also contain antioxidants and phytochemicals

that can help protect against cancer. Fiber-rich foods can also help regulate digestion and prevent constipation, which has been linked to an increased risk of colon cancer.

5. Incorporate cruciferous vegetables: Cruciferous vegetables, such as broccoli, cauliflower, kale, and Brussels sprouts, are rich in vitamins, minerals, and antioxidants that have been shown to have cancer-fighting properties. These veggies contain sulforaphane, a compound that helps the body detoxify harmful substances and may also inhibit the growth of cancer cells.

6. Stay hydrated: Drinking plenty of water is essential for overall health, but it is also important for fighting cancer. Water helps flush toxins out of the body and aids in the proper functioning of all body systems, including the immune system. Aim for at least 8 glasses of water per day, and try to limit sugary drinks as they have been linked to an increased risk of cancer.

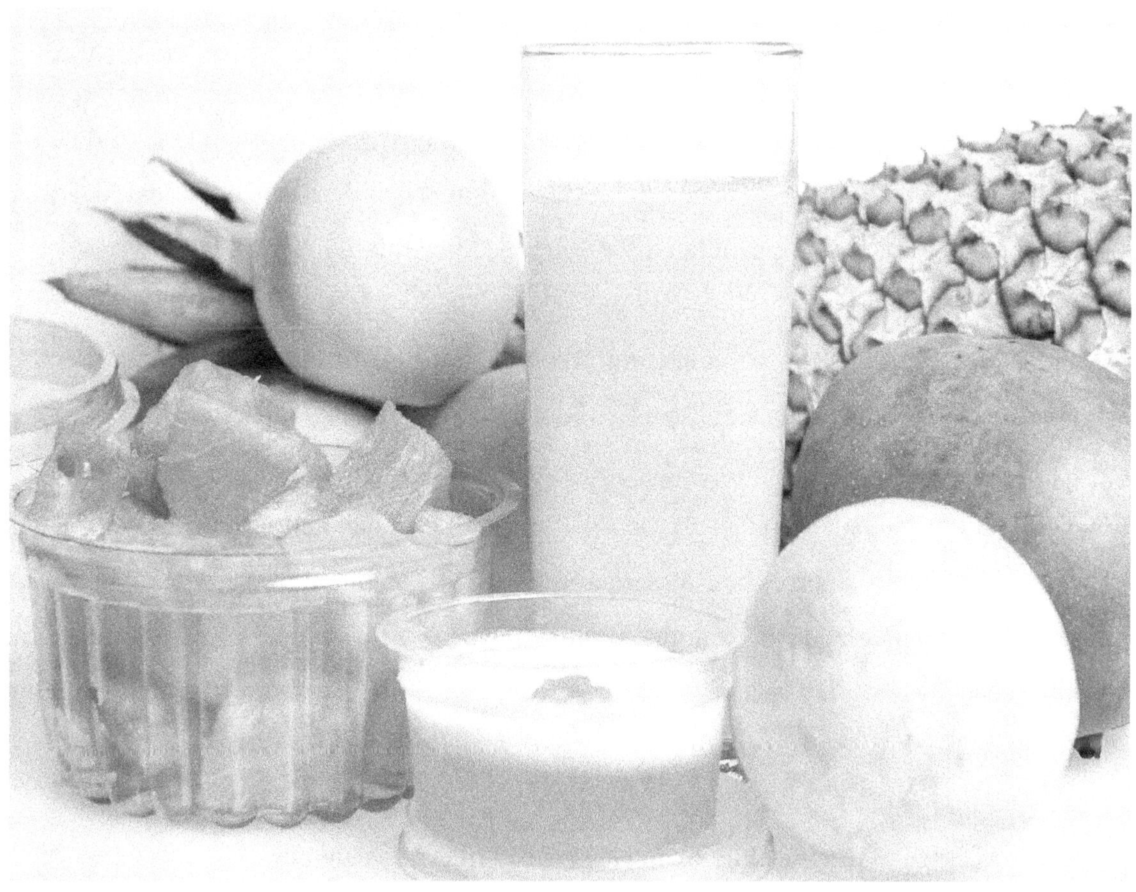

7. Limit alcohol consumption: Excessive alcohol consumption has been linked to an increased risk of several types of cancer, including breast, liver, and colon cancer. It is recommended to limit alcohol intake to no more than one drink per day for women and two drinks per day for men. In addition to following a healthy and balanced diet, here are some other important nutritional approaches to fight cancer:

- Limit added sugars: Consuming large amounts of added sugars, found in processed foods and sugary drinks, has been linked to an increased risk of cancer. Opt for whole, nutrient-dense foods instead of processed ones.

- Include probiotics and prebiotics: Probiotics are beneficial bacteria found in fermented foods like yogurt and kimchi which can help maintain a healthy gut microbiome. Prebiotics, found in foods like bananas and onions, provide food for these beneficial bacteria.

- Supplement when necessary: While a balanced diet is the best way to obtain essential nutrients, sometimes supplementation can be beneficial. Consult with a healthcare professional to determine if and what supplements may be beneficial for your specific situation.

- Avoid tobacco: Tobacco use is the leading preventable cause of cancer. Quitting smoking or using other tobacco products can significantly reduce the risk of developing cancer.

Following a healthy and balanced diet is essential for fighting cancer and supporting overall health. Along with these dietary approaches, it is also important to maintain a healthy weight, exercise regularly, and get regular health screenings. By making smart food choices and adopting a healthy lifestyle, you can significantly reduce your risk of cancer and improve your overall well-being.

Recipes For Cancer Treatment And recovery

Green Smoothie Bowl

Ingredients:

- 1 frozen banana

- 1 cup of spinach

- 1/2 cup of frozen mango

- 1/4 avocado

- 1 tbsp chia seeds

- 1 cup of almond milk

- Toppings of your choice (e.g. fresh fruits, nuts, granola)

Preparation:

1. Start by blending the frozen banana, spinach, mango, avocado, chia seeds, and almond milk together in a blender until smooth.

2. Pour the smoothie into a bowl and top it with your desired toppings.

3. Enjoy your nutritious and delicious green smoothie bowl as a breakfast or snack.

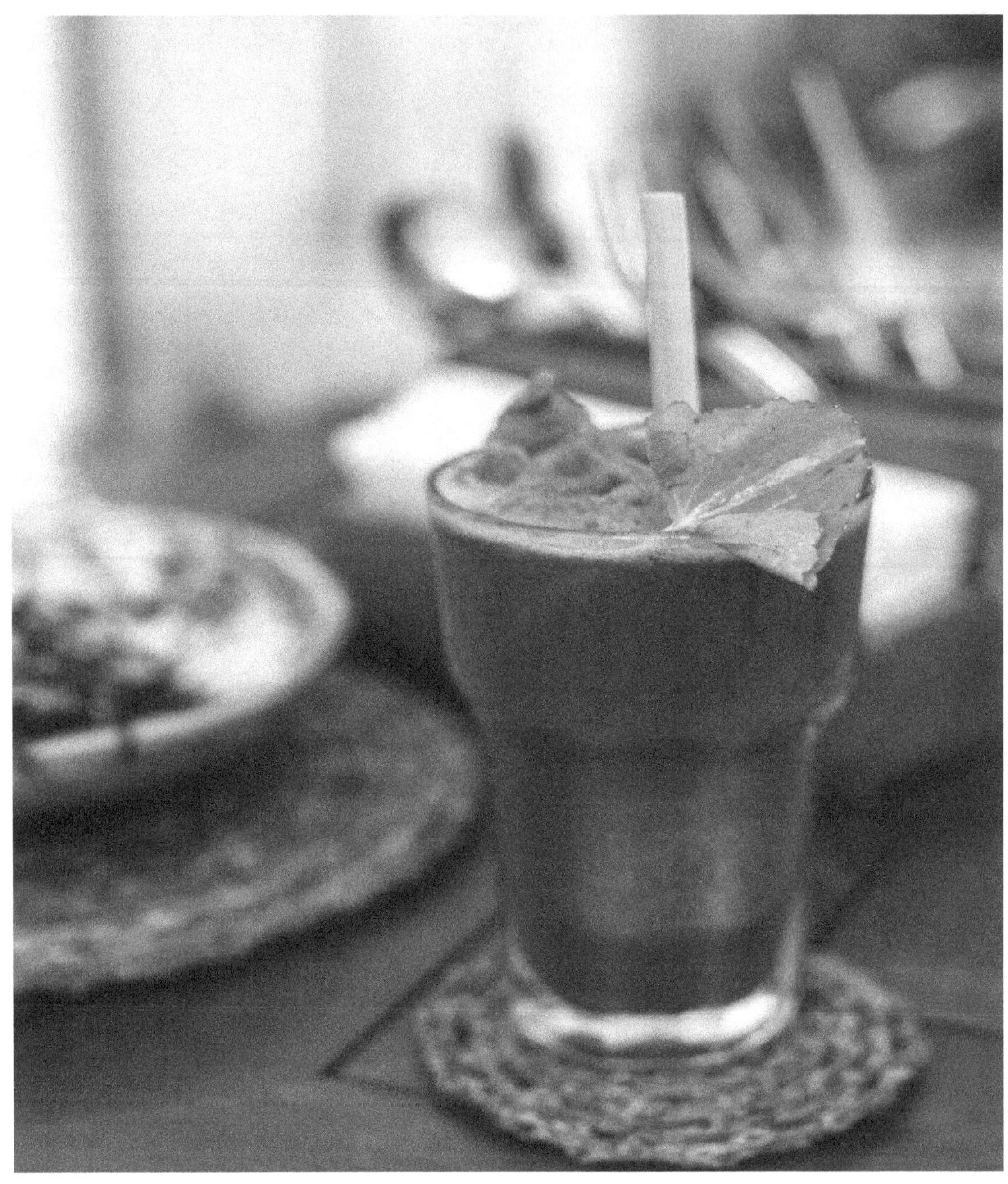

Baked Salmon with Roasted Vegetables

Ingredients:

- 4 salmon fillets

- Salt and pepper

- Garlic powder

- 1 lb of mixed vegetables (such as broccoli, bell peppers, carrots)

- Olive oil

-Fresh herbs (such as rosemary or thyme)

Preparation:

1. Preheat your oven to 375°F (190°C) and line a baking sheet with parchment paper.

2. Place the salmon fillets on the baking sheet and season them with salt, pepper, and garlic powder.

3. In a separate bowl, toss the mixed vegetables with olive oil and season with salt, pepper, and your choice of fresh herbs.

4. Spread the vegetables around the salmon fillets on the baking sheet.

5. Bake the salmon and vegetables in the oven for 15-20 minutes, until the salmon is cooked through and the vegetables are tender.

6. Serve the baked salmon with roasted vegetables on a plate and enjoy a tasty and healthy meal.

Lentil and Vegetable Soup

Ingredients:

- 1 cup green lentils

- 1 onion, chopped

- 2 garlic cloves, minced

- 2 carrots, chopped

- 2 celery stalks, chopped

- 1 can of diced tomatoes

- 4 cups vegetable broth

- 1 tsp cumin

- 1 tsp paprika

- Salt and pepper to taste

- Fresh parsley for garnish

Preparation:

1. In a large pot, heat some oil over medium heat and sauté the onion and garlic until fragrant.

2. Add in the chopped carrots and celery, and continue to cook for a few minutes.

3. Add in the lentils, diced tomatoes, vegetable broth, cumin, paprika, salt, and pepper.

4. Bring the soup to a boil, then reduce the heat and let it simmer for 20-25 minutes, until the lentils are cooked and the vegetables are tender.

5. Serve the lentil and vegetable soup in bowls and top with fresh parsley for added flavor.

Quinoa Salad: Ingredients

- 1 cup uncooked quinoa

- 1 red bell pepper, diced

- 1 cucumber, diced

- 1 avocado, diced

- 1/4 cup red onion, diced

- 1/4 cup feta cheese

- Fresh herbs (such as parsley or basil)

 For the dressing:

- 1/4 cup olive oil

- 2 tbsp lemon juice

- 1 garlic clove, minced

- Salt and pepper to taste

Preparation:

1. Rinse the quinoa and cook it according to package instructions.

2. Once the quinoa is cooked, fluff it with a fork and let it cool down.

3. In a large bowl, mix together the cooled quinoa, diced red pepper, cucumber, avocado, red onion, and feta cheese.

4. In a separate small bowl, whisk together the olive oil, lemon juice, minced garlic, salt, and pepper to make the dressing.

5. Pour the dressing over the quinoa salad and mix well.

6. Garnish with fresh herbs before serving.

Chicken and Vegetable Stir Fry

Ingredients:

- 1 lb chicken breast, cut into small cubes

- 1 tbsp oil

- Salt and pepper to taste

- 3 cups of mixed vegetables (such as broccoli, carrots, bell peppers, mushrooms)

- 1 tsp garlic powder

- 1 tsp ginger powder

- 1/4 cup soy sauce

- Cooked rice for serving

Preparation:

1. Heat oil in a large pan over medium-high heat.

2. Season the chicken cubes with salt and pepper and add them to the pan, cooking until they are fully cooked.

3. Remove the chicken from the pan and set aside.

4. In the same pan, add the mixed vegetables and cook until they are tender and slightly charred.

5. Add in the garlic powder, ginger powder, soy sauce, and cooked chicken to the pan with the vegetables, and stir fry for a few more minutes.

6. Serve the chicken and vegetable stir fry over a bed of rice and enjoy a flavorful and protein-rich meal.

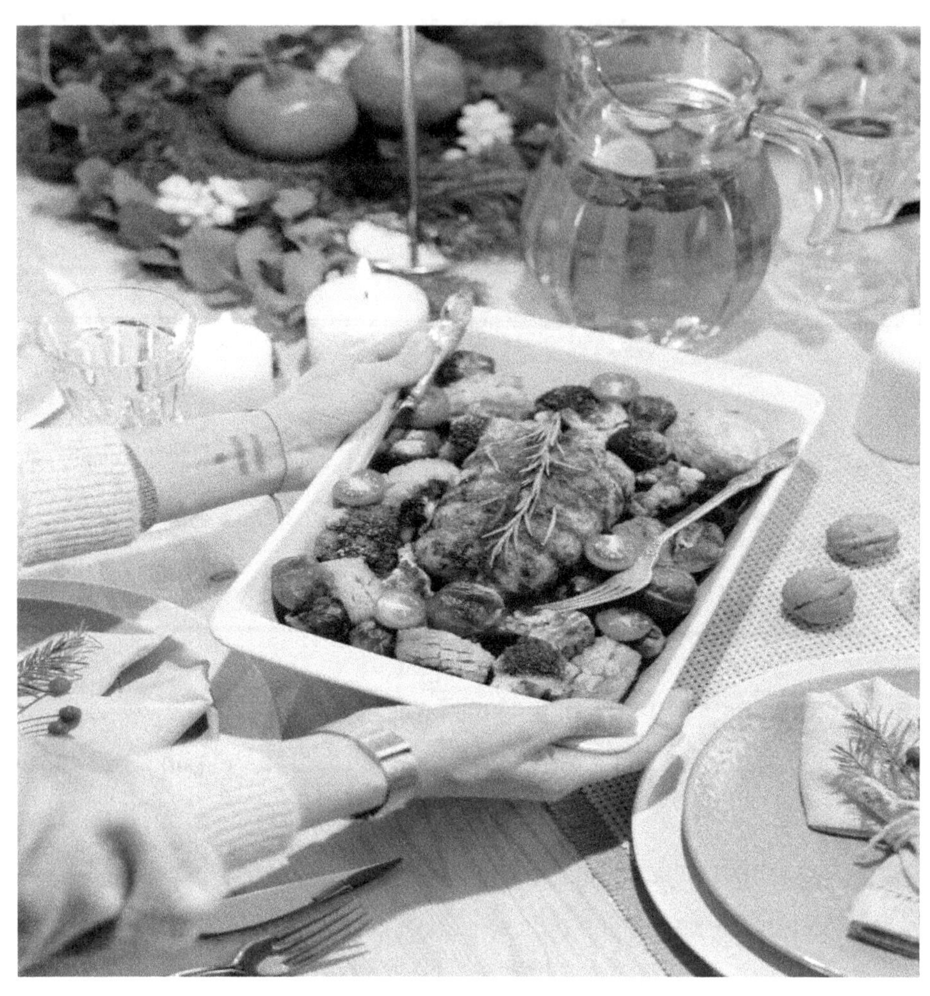

Tofu and Vegetable Curry

Ingredients:

- 1 block of firm tofu, diced

- 1 tbsp oil - Salt to taste

- 2 cloves of garlic, minced

- 1 onion, chopped

- 1 bell pepper, chopped

- 1 cup broccoli, chopped

- 1 can of coconut milk

- 2 tbsp red curry paste

- 1 tbsp soy sauce

- Cooked rice for serving

Preparation:

1. Heat oil in a large pan over medium-high heat.

2. Add in the diced tofu and cook until it is slightly browned. Season with a pinch of salt.

3. Remove the tofu from the pan and set aside.

4. In the same pan, sauté the minced garlic and chopped onion until fragrant.

5. Add in the chopped bell pepper and broccoli, and cook for a few more minutes.

6. In a separate small bowl, mix together the coconut milk, red curry paste, and soy sauce.

7. Pour the coconut milk mixture into the pan with the vegetables and stir everything together.

8. Add the tofu back into the pan and let everything simmer for 10-15 minutes.

9. Serve the tofu and vegetable curry over cooked rice for a tasty vegetarian meal.

Read more on recipes in:

Recipes for Delicious Christmas Meals by Caroline Johnson

How to starve breast cancer by Caroline Johnson

Chapter 6: Metabolic Approach To Beating Cancer

The metabolic approach to beating cancer is an alternative approach that focuses on targeting the metabolism of cancer cells to inhibit their growth and proliferation. Unlike traditional cancer treatments such as chemotherapy and radiation therapy, which primarily target rapidly dividing cells, the metabolic approach aims to starve cancer cells of the nutrients they need to survive and grow.

In order to sustain this excessive growth, cancer cells require a significant amount of energy and nutrients. This is where the metabolic approach comes in – by manipulating the metabolic processes of cancer cells, it is possible to limit their access to these vital resources and essentially "starve" them to death.

One of the key principles of the metabolic approach is the understanding that cancer cells have a distinct metabolism compared to normal cells. While healthy cells primarily use oxygen to produce energy in a process called oxidative metabolism, cancer cells rely mainly on glucose fermentation to generate energy. This means that cancer cells consume large amounts of glucose and release lactic acid as a waste product, a process known as the Warburg effect.

By understanding these metabolic differences, researchers have been able to develop various strategies to target cancer cells specifically. One example is the ketogenic diet, which is a high-fat, low-carbohydrate diet that forces the body to rely on fats for energy production instead of glucose. Since cancer cells cannot efficiently use fats as a source of energy, this diet deprives them of their main fuel source and weakens their ability to grow and divide.

Another key aspect of the metabolic approach is the use of specific supplements and drugs that can exploit the metabolic vulnerabilities of cancer cells. For example, some compounds can inhibit the activity of certain enzymes that are crucial for cancer cell metabolism. Others can interfere with signaling pathways that promote the growth and survival of cancer cells. These supplements and drugs are designed to target cancer cells specifically while leaving normal cells unharmed.

In addition to targeting the metabolism of cancer cells, the metabolic approach also focuses on optimizing the immune system to fight against cancer. A strong immune system is crucial for identifying and eliminating abnormal cells, including cancer cells. By adopting a healthy diet and incorporating immune-boosting supplements, the body's natural defense mechanisms can be strengthened to better detect and destroy cancer cells.

Furthermore, the metabolic approach recognizes the importance of reducing the burden of toxins on the body. Toxins from food, environmental pollutants, and even personal care products can accumulate in the body and contribute to the development and progression of cancer. Detoxification protocols, such as juice cleanses and saunas, can help to eliminate these toxins and support the body's natural healing processes.

The metabolic approach to beating cancer takes a holistic approach to treating the disease. It recognizes that cancer is not just a genetic or cellular aberration, but also a reflection of the overall health and lifestyle of an individual.

The metabolic approach to beating cancer is a promising alternative to traditional cancer treatments. By targeting the unique metabolism of cancer cells, this approach offers a more targeted and less toxic approach to fighting the disease. While more research is needed to fully understand its effectiveness, it has already shown promising results in certain types of cancer and has the potential to revolutionize cancer treatment in the future.

Chapter 7: Alternative Therapies And Complementary Medicines

Cancer is a disease which affects millions of people worldwide. Traditional treatments such as chemotherapy, radiation therapy, and surgery have long been the standard of care for treating cancer. However, these treatments often come with adverse side effects and may not always be effective. Alternative therapies and complementary medicines have gained popularity as potential treatments for cancer, offering patients a way to manage symptoms and side effects while also targeting the disease itself.

Some of the alternative therapies and complementary medicines that have been used in cancer treatment include herbal and botanical remedies, acupuncture, massage therapy, hypnosis, and mind-body practices like meditation and yoga. While these therapies cannot cure cancer, they can help improve overall well-being and quality of life for cancer patients by reducing pain, stress, and other side effects of traditional treatments.

Herbal and botanical remedies have been used for centuries in traditional medicine systems such as Ayurveda and Chinese medicine. Some of the herbs and plants commonly used in cancer treatment include turmeric, ginger, ginseng, and green tea. These natural remedies have shown potential in reducing inflammation, boosting the immune system, and even inhibiting the growth of cancer cells.

Acupuncture is a Chinese traditional medicine practice that has to do with the insertion of thin needles into specific points in the body to stimulate energy flow. Studies have shown that acupuncture can help reduce chemotherapy-induced nausea and vomiting, as well as pain and other symptoms in cancer patients.

Massage therapy has been found to be effective in managing pain, fatigue, anxiety, and depression in cancer patients. It involves the manipulation of soft tissues to improve circulation, reduce tension, and promote relaxation. Massage therapy can also help improve sleep and enhance overall well-being in cancer patients.

Mind-body practices, such as meditation and yoga, have gained attention for their potential benefits in relieving stress and improving mental and emotional well-being in cancer patients. These practices can help patients cope with the physical and emotional stress of their diagnosis and treatment, as well as offer a sense of control and empowerment.

While these alternative therapies and complementary medicines show promise in improving quality of life and managing side effects in cancer patients, it is important to note that they should not be used as a replacement for traditional treatments. It is crucial to consult with a healthcare professional before starting any alternative treatment to ensure that it does not interfere with prescribed medications or treatments.

Alternative therapies and complementary medicines can play a supportive role in cancer treatment by improving overall well-being, managing symptoms, and reducing side effects. While further research is still needed to determine their effectiveness in treating cancer, these therapies can

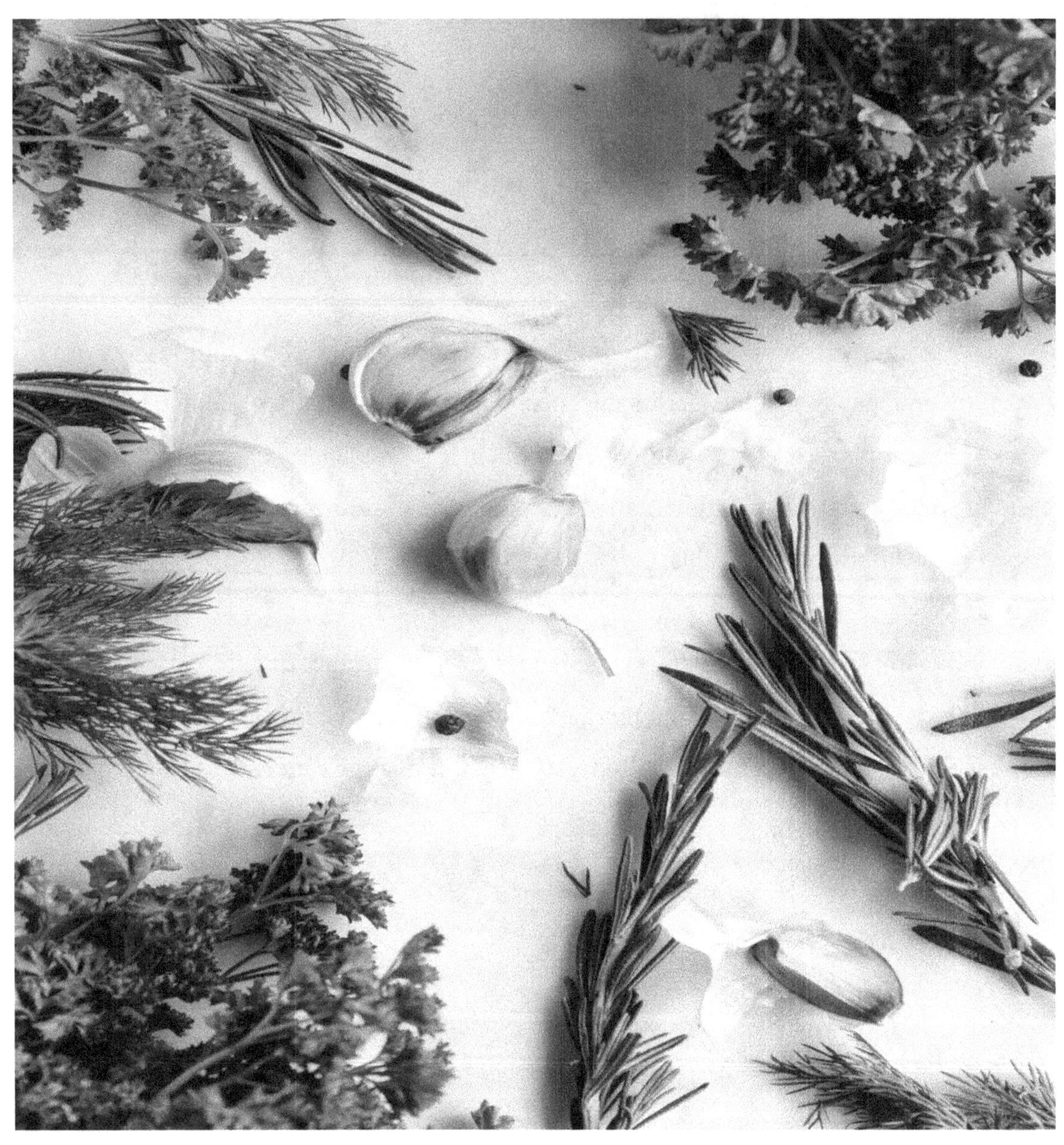

Chapter 8: Cancer And Relationships: Navigating the impact on family, friends and intimate partners.

Being diagnosed with cancer can have a profound impact on an individual's life, including their relationships with family, friends, and intimate partners. Cancer brings about physical, emotional, and social changes that can disrupt the dynamics of any relationship. Navigating this journey and its impact on loved ones requires understanding, communication, and support.

Family relationships are often the first to be affected when someone is diagnosed with cancer. Family members may experience a range of emotions, from shock and fear to sadness and guilt. They may also struggle with feeling helpless or not knowing how to support their loved one. As the patient goes through treatment, family members may have to take on new roles, such as being a caregiver, which can be emotionally and physically draining. This can lead to conflicts and strain on the relationship.

Communication is crucial in maintaining familial relationships during this time. The patient and their family members should openly discuss their feelings and concerns. It is important for family members to understand the patient's needs and preferences and to respect their decisions regarding treatment.

On the other hand, the patient should also acknowledge the physical and emotional toll that cancer takes on their loved ones. Honesty, empathy, and patience are key in navigating the impact of cancer on family relationships. Similarly, friendships can also be affected by a cancer diagnosis. Friends may struggle with finding the right words to say or may feel awkward and unsure of how to act around the patient.

Some friends may also distance themselves, either out of fear or not knowing how to support their friend. This can be hurtful for the patient, who may need emotional support from their friends during this difficult time. To navigate the impact of cancer on friendships, it is important for both the patient and their friends to communicate openly.

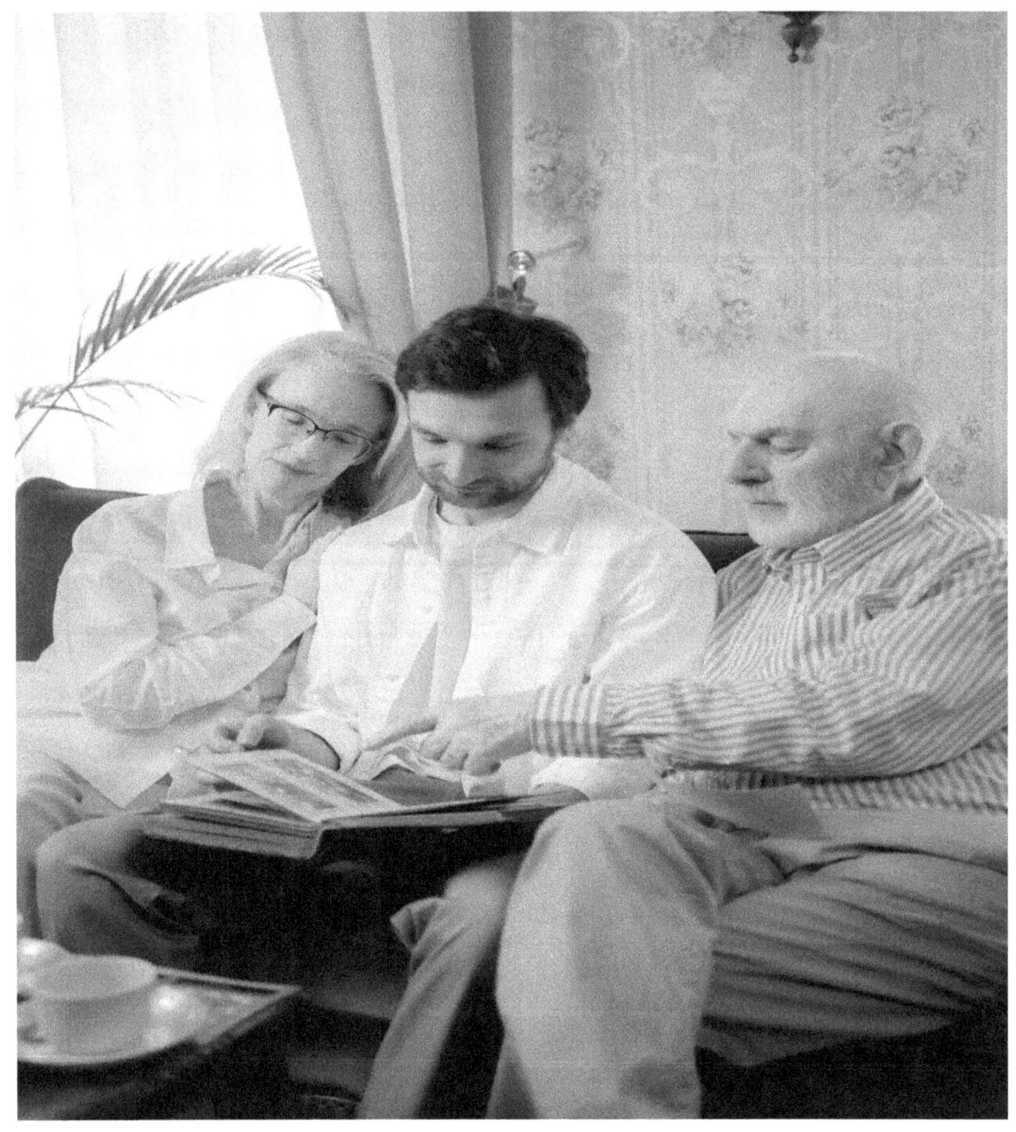

The patient may need to communicate their needs and how their friends can support them, whether it is through offering practical help or simply being there to listen. Friends should also be understanding and patient, as the patient may not have the energy to maintain the same level of communication or activities as before.

It is also important for friends to educate themselves about the patient's cancer and its treatments, so they can offer informed support. Intimate relationships can also be significantly impacted by a cancer diagnosis. Cancer treatment can cause changes in a person's physical appearance and sexual function, leading to insecurities and fears in intimate relationships. Treatments such as chemotherapy and radiation may also cause fatigue and decrease libido, making it challenging for the patient to engage in sexual activity.

Additionally, the emotional toll of cancer can also affect intimacy, as both partners may be experiencing a range of emotions. Navigating the impact of cancer on intimate relationships requires open and honest communication and understanding from both partners.

The patient may need to communicate their insecurities and concerns, and their partner should offer emotional support and reassurance. It may also be helpful for the couple to seek counseling or therapy to navigate the challenges together. Intimacy may need to take on a different form during this time, such as cuddling or spending quality time together, and partners should be understanding and patient with each other's needs.

In addition to the impact on close relationships, cancer can also affect the larger support network of the individual, including coworkers, neighbors, and acquaintances. These relationships may also experience changes as the patient may need to decrease their social activities due to treatment or may need practical support. Friends and coworkers can play a crucial role in offering support, whether it is by providing meals, running errands, or simply offering a listening ear. It is important for the patient to communicate their needs and limitations to their support network, so they can offer appropriate help. Just as importantly, the patient should also remember to thank and appreciate their support system, as it takes a village to navigate the impact of cancer.

In conclusion, cancer can have a significant impact on family, friends, and intimate relationships. Navigating this journey requires open communication, understanding, and patience from all parties involved. By acknowledging each other's needs and offering support, relationships can become even stronger during this difficult time.

Read Related books by Caroline Johnson

How to <u>Starve breast cancer</u>

<u>Teenage Sexuality</u>

Cancer Mentabolic healing

<u>Christmas Recipe</u>

Chapter 9: Caring For Yourself: Self-care and wellness during and after cancer treatment

Cancer is a debilitating disease that not only affects the body but also the mind and emotions. The journey of cancer treatment can often be overwhelming and exhausting, both physically and mentally. That's why it is crucial to prioritize self-care and focus on your overall wellness during and after cancer treatment.

Self-care is the act of taking care of oneself, both physically and mentally, to maintain good health and well-being. It involves making positive and healthy choices to improve one's quality of life. While undergoing cancer treatment, self-care might seem like a low priority, but it is vital for healing and coping with the disease.

Here are some self-care and wellness practices that can help you during and after cancer treatment:

1. Be Mindful of Your Diet: Eating a balanced and nutritious diet is essential during and after cancer treatment. The treatment often causes side effects such as nausea, loss of appetite, and changes in taste, making it challenging to maintain a healthy diet. It is crucial to focus on eating small, frequent meals rich in protein, whole grains, fruits, and vegetables to boost your immunity and energy levels.

2. Stay Physically Active: Physical activity helps to reduce the side effects of cancer treatment, such as fatigue, and can also help improve your mood and overall outlook on life. However, it is essential to consult with your doctor before starting any physical activity to ensure it is safe for you.

3. Get Adequate Rest: Cancer treatment can be physically and mentally exhausting, making it crucial to get enough rest and sleep. Listen to your body's signals, and take breaks when needed. Ensure you get at least 7-8 hours of good quality sleep each night to allow your body to heal and rejuvenate.

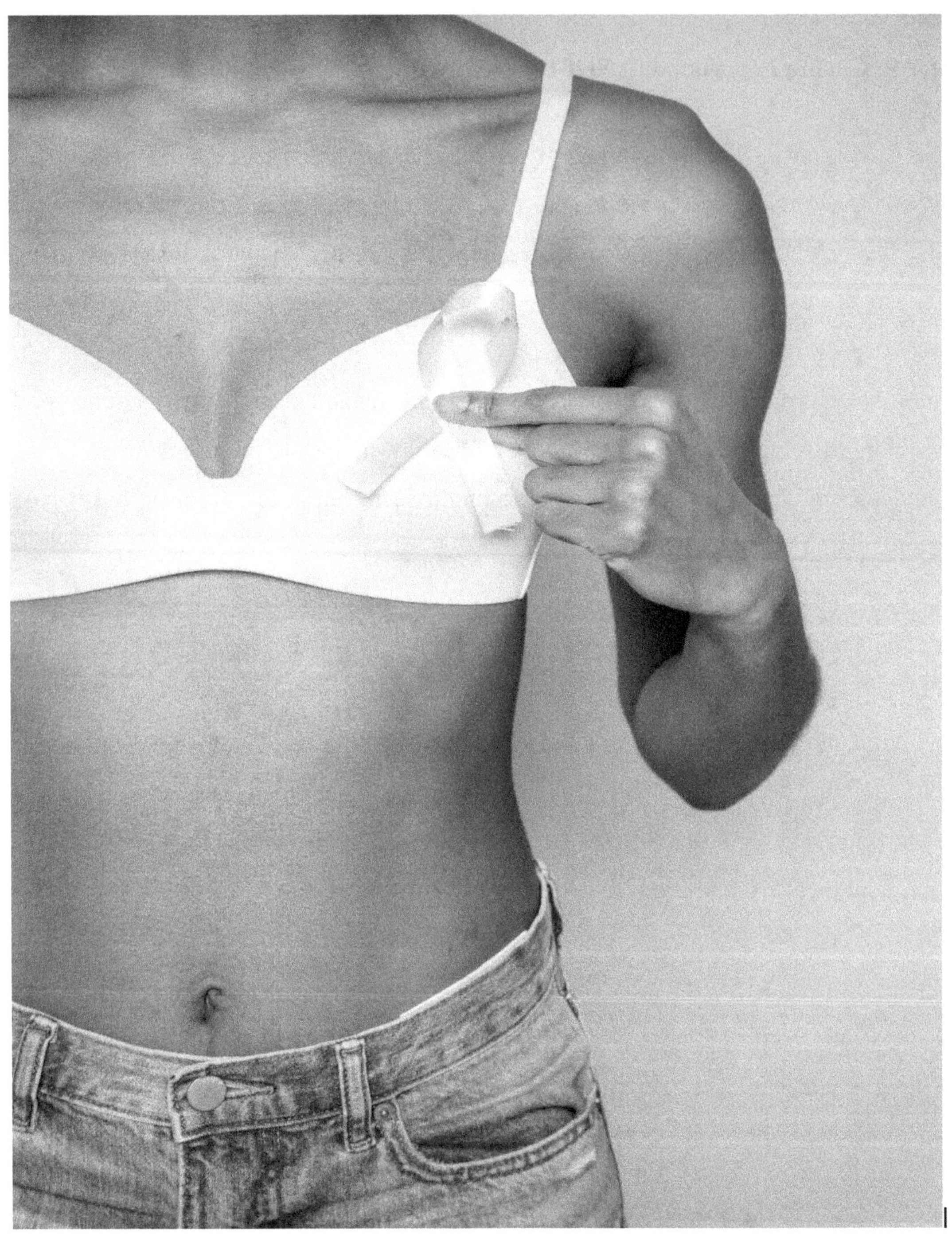

4. Practice Relaxation Techniques: Going through cancer treatment can often lead to feelings of anxiety, stress, and fear. Practicing relaxation techniques such as deep breathing, meditation, or yoga can help alleviate these feelings and promote a sense of calmness and well-being.

5. Seek Support: Don't be afraid to reach out for support from friends, family, or a support group. Having a support system can help you feel less alone in your journey and provide emotional support and assistance with practical tasks.

6. Engage in Activities that Bring You Joy: During and after cancer treatment, it is essential to engage in activities that bring you joy and make you happy. It could be something as simple as listening to music, spending time in nature, or practicing a hobby. These activities can help boost your mood, reduce stress and provide a sense of purpose.

7. Take Your Medications as Prescribed: It is crucial to follow your doctor's instructions and take your medications as prescribed. Your cancer treatment may involve several medications, and missing doses or not taking them correctly can have adverse effects on your recovery.

8. Don't Neglect Your Mental and Emotional Health: Going through cancer treatment can take a toll on your mental and emotional health. It is essential to address any feelings of depression, anxiety, or fear by seeking professional help from a mental health professional who specializes in cancer care.

9. Educate Yourself: Knowledge is power, and educating yourself about your treatment and diagnosis can help alleviate some of the fear and uncertainty. It can also help you make informed decisions about your care and communicate effectively with your healthcare team.

10. Practice Gratitude: Cancer treatment can be emotionally draining, but it's essential to remember the good things in your life. Practicing gratitude can help shift your focus from the negatives to the positives and promote a more positive mindset.

In conclusion, self-care and wellness are essential during and after cancer treatment to help you cope with the physical, emotional, and mental challenges that come with the disease. Remember to prioritize your well-being, listen to your body's needs, and seek support when needed. Taking care of yourself is not selfish; it is necessary for your healing and recovery.

Chapter 10: Support Networks and Community Resources: Finding help and support during a cancer battle

Being diagnosed with cancer can be a daunting and overwhelming experience, not only for the patient but also for their family and friends. The physical, emotional, and financial burden that comes with a cancer diagnosis can cause immense stress and anxiety. During this difficult time, it is essential to have a strong support network and access to community resources to help navigate the cancer battle.

Support networks play a crucial role in providing emotional and practical support to cancer patients. These networks can consist of family, friends, co-workers, and support groups. The love and care of family and friends can provide much-needed emotional support during this challenging time. They can lend an ear to listen, offer a shoulder to cry on, and be a source of comfort and strength. It is essential for cancer patients to reach out to their loved ones and allow them to be a part of their journey.

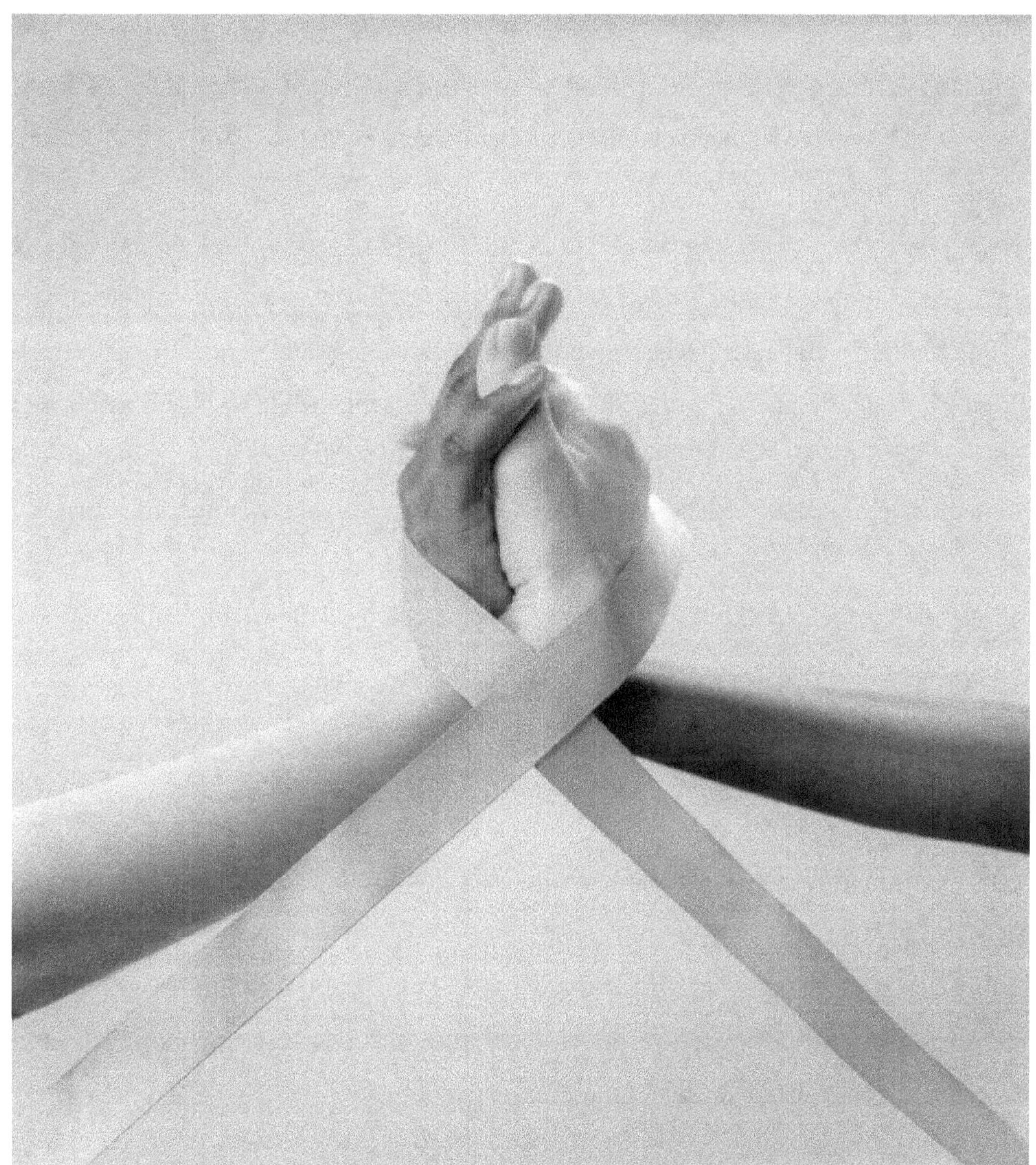

Support groups are another vital resource for cancer patients. These groups consist of individuals who are going through a similar experience and can understand the challenges and emotions that come with a cancer diagnosis. Support groups can be in-person or online, and they provide a safe space for patients to share their thoughts and feelings, seek advice and encouragement, and connect with others who truly understand their struggles. These groups offer a sense of camaraderie and support that can help alleviate the feeling of isolation that cancer patients often experience.

Aside from emotional support, support networks also play a significant role in providing practical assistance to cancer patients. This can include helping with daily tasks, such as cooking, cleaning, and running errands, or providing transportation to doctor's appointments. Having a support network that is willing to lend a helping hand can make a significant difference in a patient's day-to-day life and allow them to focus on their treatment and recovery.

In addition to support networks, accessing community resources can also be a valuable asset for cancer patients. These resources often consist of organizations and programs that offer various services, such as financial assistance, transportation, counseling, and education. These resources can help alleviate the financial burden that comes with a cancer diagnosis and provide patients with access to vital resources and information. Financial assistance programs can help cover the costs of medical treatments, medications, and other expenses related to cancer treatment.

These programs can be offered by government agencies, non-profit organizations, and charities. Patients can also receive assistance with transportation to and from medical appointments through programs such as the American Cancer Society's Road to Recovery program. Counseling and support services are also available to help cancer patients and their families cope with the emotional impact of a cancer diagnosis. These services can be found through cancer treatment centers, hospitals, and community organizations.

Counseling can provide patients with a safe space to express their emotions, learn coping mechanisms, and develop a positive mindset to face the challenges ahead. Education and information resources can also be beneficial for cancer patients.

Many organizations offer educational programs and materials that provide patients with information about their disease, treatment options, and ways to manage side effects. These resources not only empower patients to take an active role in their treatment but also help them make informed decisions about their care. A strong support network and access to community resources are crucial for cancer patients during their battle.

These resources provide much-needed emotional support, practical assistance, and access to valuable services and information. It is essential for patients to seek out these resources and allow themselves to lean on their support network during this challenging time. With the right support and resources, cancer patients can feel less alone and more empowered on their journey towards healing and recovery.

Read related books by Caroline Johnson

How to starve breast cancer

Teenage Sexuality

Recipes for delicious Christmas meals

Cancer metabolic healing

Chapter 11: Advocacy And Awareness: Taking Action for the cancer cause

Advocacy and awareness are two essential components in the fight against cancer. Cancer is a devastating disease that affects millions of people globally every year. It is a complex disease that requires multidisciplinary efforts to combat it. In addition to medical research and advancements in treatment, advocacy and awareness play a crucial role in raising public awareness, influencing policy changes, and funding for cancer research. Advocacy is the act of speaking in support of a particular cause or issue.

Cancer advocacy seeks to elevate the cancer cause and educate the public about the disease, its prevention, and treatment. It also involves influencing government policies and funding for cancer-related programs. This can be achieved through various activities such as lobbying, holding public events, and engaging with policymakers. One of the primary goals of cancer advocacy is to increase public awareness and understanding of the disease. This is crucial because many people still have misconceptions and myths about cancer, which can lead to delayed diagnosis and treatment.

By educating the public about the signs and symptoms of cancer and the importance of early detection, advocacy efforts can help reduce cancer-related mortality rates. Furthermore, advocacy is a powerful tool for influencing policies related to cancer prevention and treatment. Through advocacy, the cancer community can push for legislation that supports cancer research, improves access to affordable and quality healthcare, and promotes healthy lifestyle choices that can reduce the risk of cancer.

By working with government officials and policymakers, cancer advocates can help shape policies that are effective in combating cancer and improving the lives of those affected by the disease. Another critical aspect of advocacy for the cancer cause is fundraising. The fight against cancer requires significant financial resources, and advocates play a crucial role in raising funds for research and support programs.

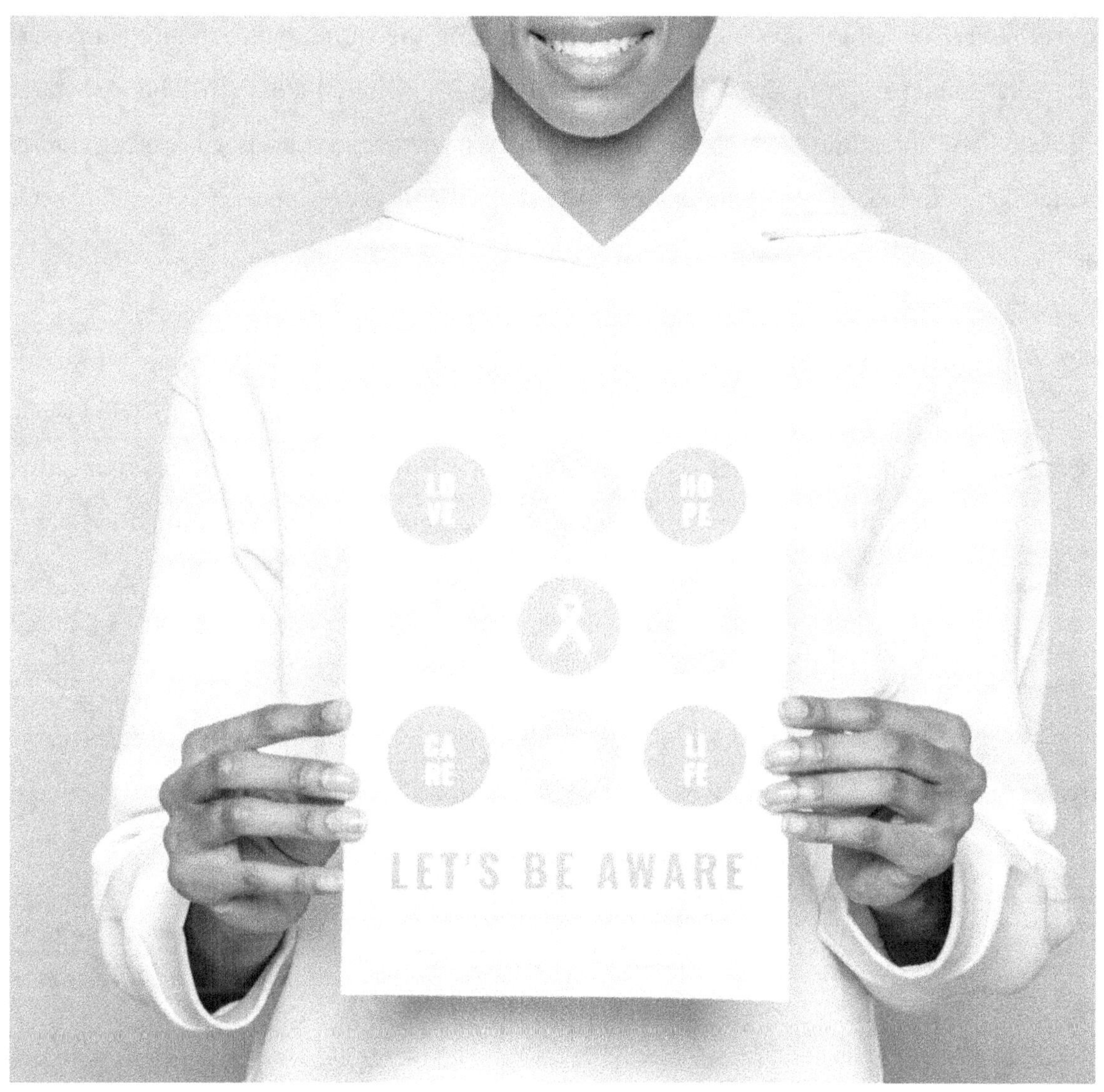

They organize various fundraising events, such as walks, runs, and galas, to generate awareness and donations for the cause. These funds are vital in supporting cancer treatment and research, as well as providing essential services to patients and their families.

In addition to advocacy, creating awareness is also crucial in the fight against cancer. While advocacy works towards systemic change, awareness-raising aims to educate individuals about the disease and promote healthy behaviors that can help prevent cancer. This involves disseminating accurate information through various channels, including social media, educational campaigns, and community outreach programs. By educating the public, people can make informed choices about their health and take steps to reduce their risk of developing cancer.

Moreover, awareness also plays a crucial role in breaking the stigma surrounding cancer. Many cancer patients and survivors face discrimination and social isolation due to misconceptions about the disease. By spreading awareness and sharing empowering stories of cancer survivors, advocates can help break the stigma and provide support and understanding to those affected by cancer.

Taking action for the cancer cause requires the collective efforts of everyone - individuals, organizations, and governments. Advocacy and awareness go hand in hand in achieving this goal. While advocacy aims to influence policies and fundraising, awareness aims to inform and empower individuals to take control of their health. Together, these two components create a powerful force in the fight against cancer.

Advocacy and awareness play a crucial role in the fight against cancer. By raising public awareness, advocating for policy changes, and fundraising for research, advocates are instrumental in advancing the cancer cause. It is imperative to continue investing our time and resources in advocacy and awareness to create a world where no one has to suffer from cancer. Together, we can make a positive impact and bring hope for a future free of cancer.

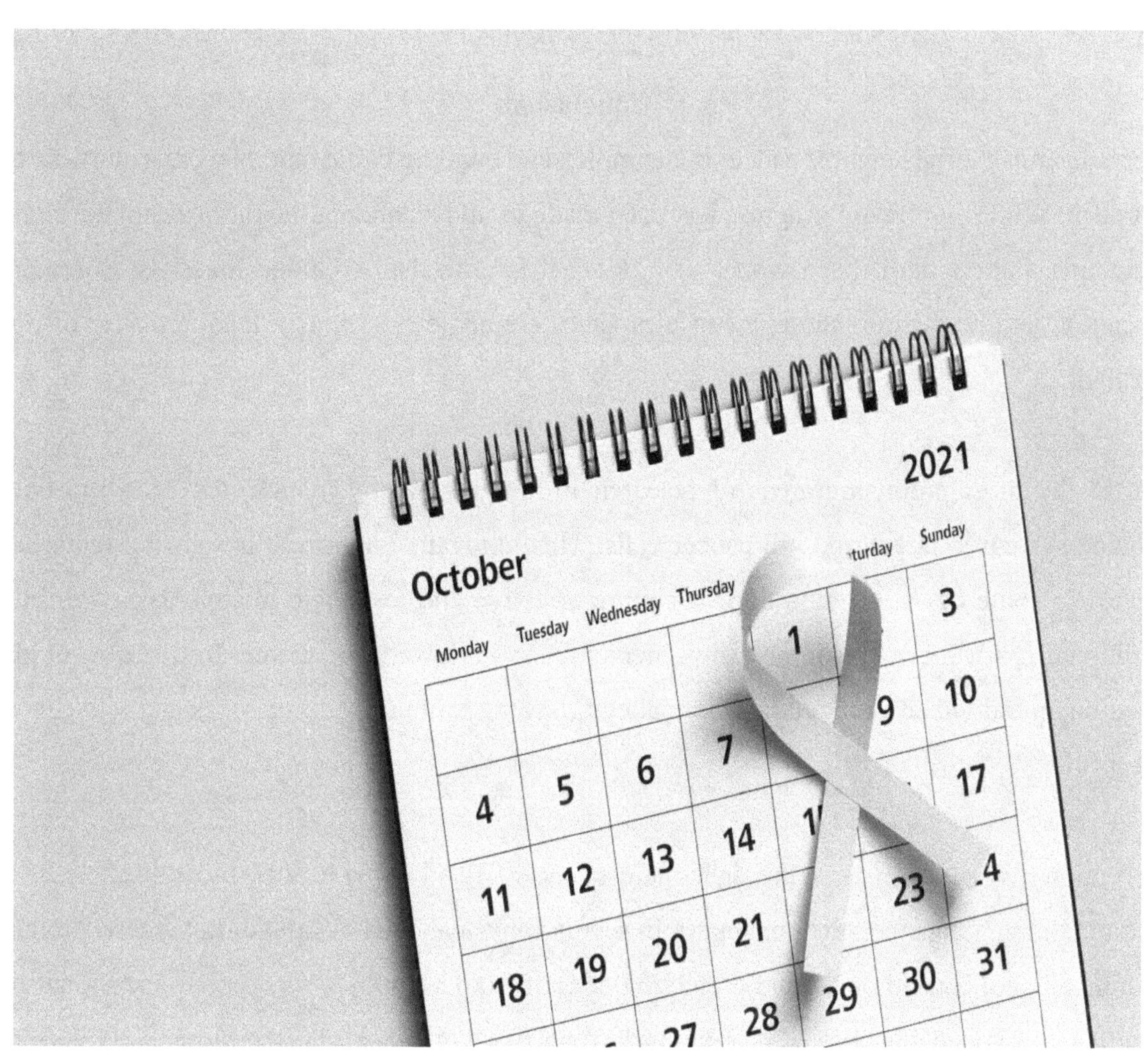

October
2021
Monday
Tuesday
Wednesday
Thursday
turday
Sunday
1
3
9
10
4
5
6
7
17
11
12
13
14
1
23
.4
18
19
20
21
29
30
31
27
28

Conclusion

In conclusion, the fight against cancer is a complex and ongoing battle that requires a multi-faceted approach. While significant progress has been made in understanding the disease and developing treatments, there is still much work to be done. It is crucial to continue investing in research, education, and prevention strategies to ultimately eliminate cancer as a leading cause of death worldwide.

One of the most promising areas of research is immunotherapy, which harnesses the body's immune system to target and kill cancer cells. This innovative approach has shown remarkable success in some cases, offering hope for more effective and less toxic treatments in the future. Additionally, advancements in precision medicine have allowed for personalized treatment plans based on an individual's unique genetic makeup, leading to improved outcomes and reduced side effects.

Prevention plays a vital role in the fight against cancer. By adopting healthy lifestyle choices such as maintaining a balanced diet, engaging in regular physical activity, avoiding tobacco products, limiting alcohol consumption, and protecting oneself from harmful UV radiation, individuals can significantly reduce their risk of developing certain types of cancer. Furthermore, early detection through regular screenings and self-examinations can lead to earlier intervention and better treatment outcomes.

Collaboration between researchers, healthcare professionals, policymakers, and advocacy groups is essential for making significant strides in cancer prevention and treatment. By sharing knowledge, resources, and expertise across disciplines and institutions, we can accelerate progress and overcome challenges more effectively.

Public awareness campaigns are crucial for educating the general population about the importance of cancer prevention and early detection. By disseminating accurate information about risk factors, symptoms, screening guidelines, and available resources, we can empower individuals to take control of their health and make informed decisions.

It is also important to address disparities in access to quality healthcare services. Cancer affects individuals from all walks of life; however, certain populations face higher rates of incidence and mortality due to factors such as socioeconomic status, race/ethnicity, and geographic location. Efforts should be made to ensure that everyone has equal access to cancer prevention, screening, and treatment options.

Furthermore, investment in cancer research is vital to drive innovation and develop new therapies. Governments, philanthropic organizations, and private sector entities should continue to allocate resources towards cancer research to support breakthrough discoveries and improve patient outcomes.

Support for cancer patients and their families is equally important. Emotional, psychological, and financial support services can help individuals navigate the challenges of a cancer diagnosis and treatment journey. By providing a holistic approach to care, we can enhance the overall well-being of patients and improve their quality of life.

In conclusion, the fight against cancer requires a comprehensive approach that encompasses prevention, early detection, innovative treatments, research advancements, public awareness campaigns, collaboration among stakeholders, addressing healthcare disparities, and support for patients. By combining these efforts, we can continue to make significant progress in the fight against cancer and ultimately strive towards a world where this devastating disease is eradicated.

Bonus

10 Days Meal Plan (well balanced diet for cancer treatment)

	Breakfast	Lunch	Dinner	Dessert
Day 1	Zucchini noodles with tomato sauce	Roasted Beet salad with walnuts	Vegan chilli with beans and vegetable	Baked apples stuffed with oat
Day 2	Green smoothie with spinach	Baked sweet potato fries	Lentil soup with tumeric and ginger	Carrot cake muffins with cream
Day 3	Vegan sushi rolls with avocado	Cauliflower crust pizza with vegetable toppings	Spaghetti squash Noddles with marinara sauce	Chai seed pudding with berries and sliced almond
Day 4	Vegan macaroni and cheese	Roasted eggplant	Carrot ginger soup topped with pumpkin seed	Banana and almond butter
Day 5	Cucumber, tomatoes and avocado salad	Vegetable curry stew and pasta	Stuffed bell peppers with quinoa and black beans	Quinoa pudding with dried apricots
Day 6	Vegan black bean bugger	Vegan pad thai with tofu and vegetables	Baked falafel wraps with tashini sauce	Fresh fruit salad with honey
Day 7	Lentil soup with tumeric and ginger	Roasted Brussels sprouts with balsamic glaze	Grilled portobello mushroom steaks	Avocado chocolate mousse
Day 8	Chickpea salad	Mushroom risotto with nutritional yeast	Roasted butternut squash soup	Grilled peach skewers

Day 9	Grilled vegetable skewers	Vegan creamy tomato pasta with cashew cream sauce	Stuffed mushrooms with quinoa spinach	Coconut milk smoothie
Day 10	Veggie sti- fry with tofu	Vegan black bean burger	Cauliflower crust pizza with vegetable toppings	Yogurt parfait with mashed banana